BUILD MUSCLE
LOSE FAT

A GET TO THE POINT
SCIENTIFIC REVIEW

STEVEN CHU

TABLE OF CONTENTS

1. Disclaimer 1

2. Introduction 2

3. Muscle & Fat... 4

4. Energy 6

5. The Secret Is Out 8

6. Establishing Baseline.. 12

7. Lose Weight 15

    7.1. Cutting Diet...17

    7.2. Cutting Macros 22

    7.3. Cutting Calculation..................................25

8. Build Muscle 29

    8.1. The Surplus 30

    8.2. Bulking Macros 32

    8.3. Bulking Calculation 34

    8.4. When To Bulk 35

9. One More Tip 40

10. Training Scheme..**42**

    10.1. Instructions 45

    10.2. The Split 48

    10.3. Deload 52

11. Supplements **55**

    11.1. Whey Protein.. 57

    11.2. Creatine.. 60

    11.3. Vitamin D... 61

    11.4. Fish Oil 63

    11.5. How To Take 64

12. Summary **69**

1. DISCLAIMER

I strongly encourage you to verify the information herein. I do my best to search for and review the literature that is relevant to the topics discussed in this book. I am not a medical doctor or self-proclaimed fitness guru. The content in this book is for informational purposes only. Although the author and publisher have made significant effort to ensure that the information in this book is correct at press time, the author and publisher do not assume and hereby disclaim any liability to any party for any loss, damage, or disruption caused by errors or omissions, whether such errors or omissions result from negligence, accident, or any other cause.

This book is not intended as a substitute for the medical advice of physicians. The reader should regularly consult a physician in matters relating to his/her health and particularly before beginning any workout program or diet or making changes to your current workout program or diet.

Nothing in this book and nothing in our statements to you should be construed as a promise or guarantee about the outcome of your fitness and health. We make no such promises or guarantees.

The reader assumes all risk, injury, loss or damage alleged to have been caused directly or indirectly by using the information presented herein.

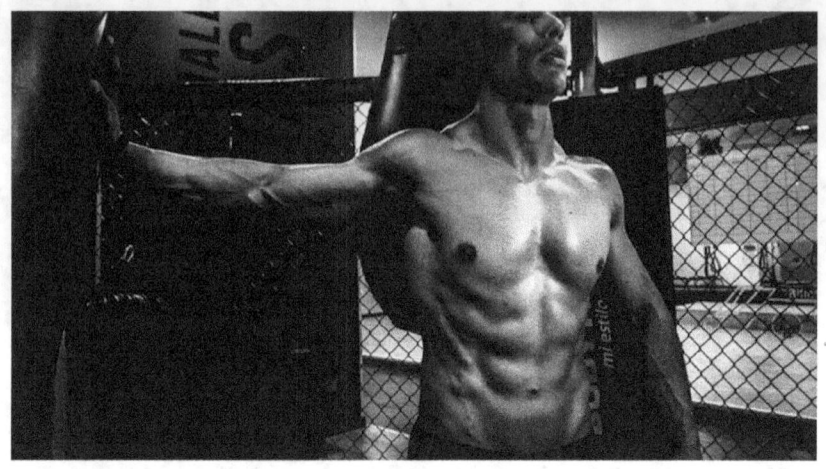

2. INTRODUCTION

Belly fat or the visceral fat that surrounds your organs, specifically the liver, heart, intestines, and stomach poses a danger to our health. Medical professionals call it metabolic syndrome; a metabolic sequelae resulting from the hormones and substances that are released by these fat cells that put you at risk for heart disease, diabetes, high blood pressure and cholesterol abnormality. Scientists recently discovered upward of 20 hormones and unidentified substances being released by these, once thought inert, fat cells (7). Muscles, on the other hand, do the opposite of fat. Muscles are metabolically active in removing sugar from your blood, reducing inflammation, and assisting in fat burning. Resistance training can help build muscles to counteract against the danger of body fat. For those of you who are ready to reduce your risks of the metabolic syndrome, but you don't know where to start because the information on how to train, as well as how to eat is overwhelmingly confusing. You want to take supplements to help accelerate your progress, but the options are endless and you just don't have the budget to buy them all. Well, you have come to the right place. I will simplify that process for you by providing you with real, unbiased scientific findings regarding the best strategies to build muscle and lose body fat, what to eat and how much, and which supplements to take to augment your training and nutrition. I will not try to sell you supplements or special training regimen that promises never before seen results. Without further ado, let's start!

3. MUSCLE & FAT

Muscle growth is a desirable goal. Muscles counteract the negative consequences of fat and the metabolic syndrome that accompanies it. Muscles also enhance athletic performance which can translate to functional performance in real life like lifting a box, playing with your kids and doing chores. Our growth potential is determined by our genetics and training experience (3). It is commonly accepted that a positive energy balance is in itself a stimulus for muscle growth, but when coupled with strength training, muscle growth is optimized (4). A positive energy balance occurs when the energy we consume, whether it is from solid foods or drinks, exceeds the energy we expend or burn via activities. Keep in mind that bodily processes, such as digestion, thinking, memorizing, etc., also expend energy. On the other hand, if the energy balance is negative, which means that energy coming in falls below energy used, then we lose both lean and fat mass. This is what is referred to as Calories In vs. Calories Out. We now know that energy balance is an important determinant of which direction the needle on the scale will move. Nutrition and training are two important factors in the building of muscle and/or losing fat. Can we gain muscle and lose fat at the same time or are they two different processes that must be done separately? Do we need to cycle between phases of bulking and cutting? How should we approach nutrition and training to achieve these two goals? Let's examine nutrition in more details, what is energy and how do we determine how much energy is needed for each person. Our goal is to come up with a nutritional plan and weight training program that maximizes muscle gain coupled with fat loss.

4. ENERGY

We obtain our energy from the calories that are stored in our foods and drinks, which also contain macronutrients that our body is unable to make. These macronutrients are protein, carbohydrate, and fat. Protein is broken down into amino acids, which are building blocks for many things, but we are only interested in muscle for the scope of this book.

Recently, we know that protein is important for body composition as well. For example, when subjects of a study consumed a high amount of protein than that of the U.S. Recommended Dietary Allowance (RDA), Antonio et al. saw an increase in lean body mass and reduction in fat mass (6). Carbohydrate is broken down into glucose, which is the preferred source of energy. The excess glucose that is not utilized immediately is converted to glycogen to be stored away in mostly the liver and muscle, or into adipose tissues to be stored in fat cells to be used later in the event that the body is low on glucose. Fats have vital functions, such as assisting in the absorption of vitamins and minerals, maintenance of body temperature, healthy skin, cell walls, and help keep hormones in balance. There are good and bad fats. You should avoid trans-fats, while mono- and polysaturated fats are considered "good" fats. The take home point is that each one of these macronutrients have its roles and functions. You simply cannot avoid either one long-term without suffering some form of consequences. That's why on this plan you will never have to avoid any food group. We will explore the appropriate macronutrients ratio that will allow us to build muscle and reduce fat as optimally as possible, while minimizing any long-term effects.

Our objectives are three folds. The first objective is to individualize each person's energy balance and formulate a macronutrients ratio that will allow us to build muscle and lose fat, if that is possible. The second objective is to design a training program that will augment our nutritional strategy to increase strength, lean mass and reduce fat mass according to each individual's training experience. Lastly, we want to use supplements, if they truly are beneficial, to help us reach our goals. We will apply scientific findings to each of these goals. We will not be using anecdotal evidences in our program. In fact, we aim to refute such anecdotal claims that are not backed by concrete research data. We will make continuous improvements to this book as new data become available, but only if they are reliable, irrefutable and replicable data.

5. THE SECRET IS OUT

It is quite simple, isn't it? If you want to gain weight, eat more to create a caloric surplus. If you want to lose weight, eat less and/or move more to create a caloric deficit. It is all about *Calories In vs. Calories Out* (1). So, is this all you need to build muscle or lose fat? It is more complicated than that, of course. We are under two assumptions here. The first is that if we eat a caloric surplus, then the weight we gain is purely muscle. The second assumption, on the opposite end of the spectrum, is that if we eat a caloric deficit, then the weight we lose is purely fat. I am sure you already sensed something is wrong with such assumptions. Indeed, these assumptions cannot be further from the truth. Why?

When you are in a caloric surplus, your body can utilize either protein and carbohydrates to make muscle, aka muscle protein synthesis. It can also make fat from the excess glucose. Our body doesn't discriminate and give us what we want, which is to make more muscles than fat. In other words, when in a caloric surplus, we gain both muscles and fat.

When you are in a caloric deficit, you guessed it...our body will burn both fat and muscles (2). Furthermore, when we are in a calorie-restricted diet, our body is essentially in a catabolic (breakdown) state. Building muscles is an anabolic (synthesis) state. These are two antagonizing states. Yet, the Antonio et al. study noted above proved otherwise. You can indeed gain muscle and lose fat at the same time (6). We just need to find out the conditions that allowed for these two, seemingly separate, processes to occur simultaneously. We will explore more proofs that it is possible to build muscles and lose fat at the same time.

REFERENCES

1. Romieu I, Dossus L, Barquera S, Blottière HM, Franks PW, Gunter M, Hwalla N. (2017). "Energy balance and obesity: what are the main drivers?" Cancer Causes & Control 28 (3):247-258.

2. Helms ER, Aragon AA, Fitschen PJ. (2014). Evidence-based recommendations for natural bodybuilding contest preparation: nutrition and supplementation. Journal of the International Society of Sports Nutrition, 11:20.

3. Garthe I, Raastad T, Refsnes PE, Sundgot-Borgen J. (2013). Effect of nutritional intervention on body composition and performance in elite athletes. European Journal of Sport Science, 13 (3): 295-0303, http://dx.doi.org/10.1080/17461391.2011.643923.

4. Rozenek R, Ward P, Long S, Garhammer J. (2002). Effects of high- calorie supplements on body composition and muscular strength following resistance training. Journal of Sports Medicine and Physical Fitness, 42: 3400-347.

5. Hall, K. (2008). What is the Required Energy Deficit per unit Weight Loss? Int J Obes (Lond) , 32 (3), 573-576.

6. Antonio J. (2014). The effects of consuming a high protein diet (4.4 g/kg/d) on body composition in resistance-trained individuals. JISSN , 11 (19).

7. Rosenow A, Arrey TN, Bouwman FG, Noben JP, Wabitsch M, Mariman ECM, Karas M, Renes J. Identification of novel human adipocyte secreted proteins by using SGBS cells. J Proteome Res. (2010); 9(10): 5389-5401.

6. ESTABLISHING BASELINE

We talked about how *Calories In vs. Calories Out* directly impacts our weight. The next logical step is to figure out our maintenance calories, or the total daily amount of calories that we can consume without affecting our weight. This is the amount of calories where calories in is equal to calories out. This is known as the Total Daily Energy Expenditure (TDEE). Your TDEE depends on your daily activity level and exercise intensity. As such it is still an estimate. The easiest way to calculate your TDEE would be to search for a TDEE calculator online. You can use any of them, as long as the calculator takes into account your daily activity level. Another method I would like to use is to multiply your weight in pounds by 14-17. For example, for a 170 pounds person, the TDEE would be between (170 x 14) 2380 calories and (170 x 17) 2890 calories. At the lower end of the estimate, your activity level and/or exercise intensity are low, whereas at the upper end of the estimate your activity level and/or exercise intensity are high.

Now that you know your baseline TDEE, you can consume up to this amount of calories. How do you know how many calories are in your foods? There are no easy ways to do this, except for accurately weighing your foods and tracking it using an app. The most popular foods tracking apps are MyfitnessPal, MyPlate and Lifesum. It is extremely important that you log everything. It needs to be accurate and complete. I cannot stress this enough. Be accurate and complete!

The next step is to eat up to your TDEE every day for 2 weeks. You need to weigh yourself every day at the same time every day for the next two weeks, preferably in the morning upon waking up and after going to the bathroom. Log your weight and take the average every week. You should be able to see if you are gaining weight, losing weight or no change. Here is an example:

Day 1: 170 pounds	Day 8: 169 pounds
Day 2: 172 pounds	Day 9: 173 pounds
Day 3: 169.5 pounds	Day 10: 171.2 pounds
Day 4: 171 pounds	Day 11: 169.2 pounds
Day 5: 173 pounds	Day 12: 169.6 pounds
Day 6: 169.4 pounds	Day 13: 173 pounds
Day 7: 171 pounds	Day 14: 169.3 pounds

Week 1 (Days 1-7) Average =
(170+172+169.5+171+173+169.4+171) / 7 days = 170.8 pounds

Week 2 (Days 8-14) Average =
(169+173+171.2+169.2+169.6+173+169.3) / 7 days =170.6 pounds

In this example, your weight remains the same. So, you can be sure that your estimated TDEE was accurate. Don't worry, if it is not. Proceed next to your goal of either *Lose Weight* or *Build Muscle* in the next sections. The daily fluctuations in weight might be more prominent than the example above. It is important to take the average of your weight every week for at least two weeks before you make any changes to your diet. You don't want to make drastic cuts or additional calories intake, as you can see why in the next section. Slow progress is good progress.

7. LOSE WEIGHT

Now that you know your TDEE, all you have to do is to create a caloric deficit by either consuming less or burning more through exercise or activities. Even if your TDEE estimate is not accurate in the previous section, *Establishing Baseline,* you can still lose weight by reducing your consumption. I will refer to losing weight as *cutting,* since this is the term used in the fitness world. The question is how much should you cut and for how long?

As a general rule, every pound is approximately 3500 calories. To lose one pound of fat per week, you would have to cut 500 calories from your TDEE every day, 500 calories/day x 7 days = 3500 calories or one pound of weight loss per week (1). As we discussed previously, we don't just lose fat when cutting, we also lose lean body mass. This is often the problem with a large caloric deficit. The larger the deficit, the larger the lean body mass loss (1,2,3). Garthe et al. did an experiment in which one group of athletes was assigned to lose weight at a rate of about two pounds of their body weight per week and another group at about one pound of their body weight per week. The group that lost weight at the slower rate (one pound per week) lost more fat mass, while the faster weight loss group (two pounds per week) lost less fat mass and also lost lean body mass at the same time (2). In another study by Mero et al., a weekly weight loss of 1 kg (2.2

pounds) was compared to 0.5 kg (1.1 pound) weight loss. The 1 kg weekly weight loss group had a 5% decrease in bench press strength (4).

Newton et al. did a similar study that showed a weekly weight loss of 0.5- 1% of body weight was better than faster rate at retaining lean body mass (5). When cutting, the slower the rate of weight loss and smaller the deficit, the better you will be at retaining lean body mass.

7.1. CUTTING DIET

The U.S. Recommended Dietary Allowance (RDA) guideline currently states that for most of the general population 0.8 gram/kg per day of proteins, 50% of total dietary calories for carb, and about 20-35% of total dietary calories for fats are sufficient (6).

In a study, subjects were either consuming 0.8 g/kg of proteins or 1.6 g/kg per day while in a calorie-reduced diet, the higher protein consumption group had less lean body mass loss compared to the lower protein consumption group (7). In a different study by Mettler et al., subjects diet was changed so that fats was reduced to allow for higher protein consumption of up to 2.3 g/kg/day (8). The result of the study showed that at this amount of protein consumption only a small amount of lean body mass was lost over a one week period. Yet, in another study by Helms et al. shows a range of protein consumption between 2.3-3.1 g/kg of lean body mass is optimal for lean body mass retention for athletes who are in a caloric deficit. The leaner one becomes and the larger the deficit, the higher the protein intake is necessary to retain lean body mass during cutting (9).

Carbohydrates help fuel athletic performance. Inadequate intake can impair training and glycogen restoration (10). In a study that compared a diet that reduced proteins for higher carbs and increased proteins for lower carbs, the latter group retained more lean body mass, but suffered in performance (7). Mettler et al. found that a diet with reduced fat, higher proteins and adequate carbs was superior at maintaining lean body mass and strength performance in subjects who were in a caloric deficit (8).

Dietary fat is, therefore, reduced to compensate for higher proteins and carbs consumption when cutting. However, dietary fats have been linked to hormonal balance, specifically testosterone. So, how much can we cut fat without impairing testosterone? Hämäläinen et al. switched study subjects from a diet of 40% fat to 20% fat. What they found was that the subjects' testosterone level dropped when switched to the lower fat diet. Their testosterone levels returned to normal when they were switched back to the 40% fat diet (11). Belanger et al. did a similar study and also had similar results (12). However, when looking at these studies, the subjects were consuming more polyunsaturated fats when switched to the lower fat diet. Interestingly, Tegelman et al. did a study in which subjects had reduced fat consumption, while carbohydrates consumption was increased slightly. What they found was that testosterone levels were not affected negatively when carbohydrates intake was increased in conjunction with the lower fat intake (13). A review by Lambert et al. also suggested that the interaction between low fat diet and testosterone level is a complex one and might be dependent on the type of fats consumed (14). If you are consuming a high amount of polyunsaturated commonly found in soybean oil, canola oil, sunflower seed oil, cottonseed oil, fish and margarine, it might be a good idea to keep your fat consumption higher.

The Institute of Medicine's Acceptable Macronutrient Distribution Range (AMDR) for fat intake is between 20 to 35% of total dietary calories for adults age 19 and older (6). Lambert et al.

also recommended fat intake around 15-20% of total dietary calories. In the setting of a caloric deficit, it might be prudent to keep fat intake at 20% to allow for a higher protein and carbohydrates consumption for lean body mass preservation without compromising testosterone level.

REFERENCES

1. Hall KD: What is the required energy deficit per unit weight loss? Int J Obes 2007, 32:573–576.

2. Garthe I, Raastad T, Refsnes PE, Koivisto A, Sundgot-Borgen J: Effect of two different weight-loss rates on body composition and strength and power-related performance in elite athletes. Int J Sport Nutr Exerc Metab 2011, 21:97–104.

3. Forbes GB: Body fat content influences the body composition response to nutrition and exercise. Ann N Y Acad Sci 2000, 904:359–365.

4. Mero AA, Huovinen H, Matintupa O, Hulmi JJ, Puurtinen R, Hohtari H, KarilaT: Moderate energy restriction with high protein diet results in healthier outcome in women. J Int Soc Sports Nutr 2010, 7:4.

5. Newton LE, Hunter GR, Bammon M, Roney RK: Changes in psychological state and self-reported diet during various phases of training incompetitive bodybuilders. J Strength Cond Res 1993, 7:153– 158.

6. USDA "2015–2020 Dietary Guidelines for Americans, 8th edn" (2015).

7. Walberg JL, Leidy MK, Sturgill DJ, Hinkle DE, Ritchey SJ, Sebolt DR: Macronutrient content of a hypoenergy diet affects nitrogen retention and muscle function in weight lifters. Int J Sports Med 1988, 9:261–266.

8. Mettler S, Mitchell N, Tipton KD: Increased protein intake reduces lean body mass loss during weight loss in athletes. Med Sci Sports Exerc 2010,42:326–337.

9. Helms ER, Zinn C, Rowlands DS, Brown SR: A systematic review of dietary protein during caloric restriction in resistance trained lean athletes: a case for higher intakes. Int J Sport Nutr Exerc Metab 2013.

10. Haff GG, Koch AJ, Potteiger JA, Kuphal KE, Magee LM, Green SB, Jakicic JJ: Carbohydrate supplementation attenuates muscle glycogen loss during acute bouts of resistance exercise. Int J Sport Nutr Exerc Metab 2000,10:326–339.

11. Hämäläinen EK, Adlercreutz H, Puska P, Pietinen P: Decrease of serum total and free testosterone during a low-fat high-fibre diet. J Steroid Biochem1983, 18:369–370.

12. Bélanger A, Locong A, Noel C, et al. Influence of diet on plasma steroids and sex hormone-binding globulin levels in adult men. J Steroid Biochem. 1989;32(6):829-833.

13. Tegelman R, Aberg T, Pousette A, Carlström K. Effects of a diet regimen on pituitary and steroid hormones in male ice hockey players. Int J Sports Med. 1992;13(5):424-430.

14. Lambert CP, Frank LL, Evans WJ: Macronutrient considerations for the sport of bodybuilding. Sports Med 2004, 34:317–327.

7.2. CUTTING MACROS

In a study by Layman et al., different macros ratios and exercise were compared to see their effects on body composition over 16 weeks. The objective of this study was to investigate how high protein or high carb diets affect body composition and lipid profile. We will discuss only body composition in this book. Macros profile for the high carbohydrates groups was 0.8 g/kg/ day for protein, 30% fat, carb:protein ratio > 3.5. On the other hand, the high protein groups macros profile was 30% protein, 30% fats, carb:protein ratio < 1.5. Exercise consisted of resistance training two times a week. What the researchers found was that high protein consumption preserved lean body mass and reduced body fat. The effects appeared to be additive in the presence of exercise, since the researchers also compared high protein with high protein plus exercise in this study (1).

Wycherley et al. did a similar study, but with a different diet composition and subjects in this study did resistance training 5 days a week. The carb:protein:fat ratios were 53:19:26 (no calorie deficit) vs. 43:33:22 (caloric deficit). The researchers also found favorable lean body mass preservation in the high protein group during calorie restriction, and the addition of resistance training produced more total weight loss than diet alone (2). Can protein be pushed even higher? In a study by Antonio et al., subjects were taking in as high as 4.4 g/kg/day of protein. In this study, lean or fat mass was found to be unchanged (5). In a followup study by Antonio et al., subjects were consuming 3.4 g/kg/day of protein, but training was also changed to a progressive, body-split schedule of heavy lifting with the aim to increase strength. The result was different this time. The higher protein consumption group gained lean mass and lost body fat (6).

When trying to reduce body fat and calorie restriction is necessary, keep your macronutrients consumption at 20% fat, 3.4 g/kg/day of protein, and the rest are carbohydrates. Keep in mind that as your body fat percentage gets low, you might need even higher protein intake (3).

However, the body fat percentage cutoff point is unclear for even higher protein requirement. One of the hallmark signs of lean body mass loss is loss of strength. If you find yourself in this situation, you can increase your protein intake up to 4.4 g/kg/day. If you still lose strength after increasing your protein, you can take a break from your caloric deficit by consuming up to your TDEE, but never exceed it. You can use the conventional or RDA macros ratio of 20:50:30 for protein, carb, and fat, respectively. After a few days or a week, you can go back to reduce your calories and the macros ratio above of 20% fat, 3.4 g/kg/day of protein and the rest for carbohydrates. It is possible that you will gain weight and some fat back while on your diet break. It will be negligible though, if you keep your total daily dietary calories within your TDEE. Remember weight gain or loss is dependent on total daily energy intake or calories in vs. calories out (4).

You may take a break longer than 1 week, but remember that the longer your diet break, the more weight or fat you might gain back. It should be short enough to prevent too much weight gain, while long enough to allow your body to reset. Let your strength and how you feel dictate how long you should take a break. I find one week is usually sufficient based on my own experience.

7.3. CUTTING CALCULATION

Let's now try to calculate our macros based on the above ratio and a hypothetical individual who is a 35 years old male, 170 pounds, 5'5", moderately active and moderate exercise intensity. After plugging these values into the TDEE calculator above, I got a TDEE of 2700. You can also multiply weight in pound by 14-17 to estimate TDEE. In this case, since the person is moderately active and exercise intensity is moderate, you can multiply weight in pounds by 15-16, in which case the TDEE is in the range of 2550-2720 calories. For our practice, let's go with 2700 calories as the TDEE. Rememeber to see how accurate this estimation is, weigh yourself every day for at least two weeks and calculate the average weight each week to see where you are trending, whether you are losing or gaining weight with the amount of foods consumed.

Here are some numbers to remember:

1 pound = 2.2 kg
1 gram of protein = 4 calories
1 gram of carb = 4 calories
1 gram of fat = 9 calories

Let's calculate our hypothetical case!

We want to create a 500 calories deficit up to 30% of your TDEE per day (7). For our example, let's go with a 500 calories deficit. Our TDEE is 2700 calories. So, our total daily dietary calories = 2700-500 = 2200 calories.

Fat = 2200 calories x (20/100) = 440 calories
Convert fat to grams: 440 calories / (9 calories/g) = 49 grams

Protein = (3.4 g/kg/day) x (170 pounds/2.2 kg/pound) = 263 grams
Convert protein to calories: 263 grams x (4 calories/g) = 1052 calories

Carb = 2200 calories - (440 calories + 1052 calories) = 708 calories
Convert carb to grams: 708 calories / (4 calories/g) = 177 grams

So, you would consume 263 grams of protein, 177 grams of carb and 49 grams of fat. The final step would be to track everything you eat or drink that contain calories. Try to consume as close to these macros as possible. Buy yourself a food scale to weigh your foods. It is advisable that you weigh your food prior to cooking. Cooked food loses weight and size and you might end up over-consuming without realizing it. For example, a six ounce chicken breast might shrink to four ounces when cooked. So, if you weigh out six ounces of cooked chicken breast, you might inadvertently consume nine ounces of cooked chicken instead. This is a huge problem, if you are trying to lose weight. The bottom line is try to consume as close to these macros and calories as possible.

REFERENCES

1. Layman DK, Boileau RA, Erickson DJ, Painter JE, Shiue H, Sather C, Christou DD: A reduced ratio of dietary carbohydrate to protein improves body composition and blood lipid profiles during weight loss in adult women. J Nutr 2003, 133:411–417.

2. Wycherley TP, Noakes M, Clifton PM, Cleanthous X, Keogh JB, Brinkworth GD: A High-Protein Diet With Resistance Exercise Training Improves Weight Loss and Body Composition in Overweight and Obese Patients With Type 2 Diabetes. Diabetes Care 2010, 33:969-976.

3. Eric R Helms, Alan A Aragon and Peter J Fitschen. Evidence-based recommendations for natural bodybuilding contest preparation: nutrition and supplementation. Journal of the International Society of Sports Nutrition 2014, 11:20.

4. Jakicic, J. M., Clark, K., Coleman, E., Donnelly, J. E., Foreyt, J., Melanson,E. L., Volek, J., Volpe, S. L. & American College of Sports Medicine (2001). American College of Sports Medicine position stand. Appropriate interventionstrategies for weight loss and prevention of weight regain for adults. Med. Sci.Sports Exerc. 33: 2145–2156.

5. Antonio J. (2014). The effects of consuming a high protein diet (4.4 g/kg/d) on body composition in resistance-trained individuals. JISSN , 11 (19).

6. Antonio J, A. E. (2015). A high protein diet (3.4 g/kg/d) combined with a heavy resistance training program improves body composition in healthy trained men and women – a follow-up investigation. JISSN , 12 (39).

7. Pasiakos SM, Cao JJ, Margolis LM, Sauter ER, Whigham LD, McClung JP, Rood JC, Carbone JW, Combs JF, and Young AJ. Effects of high- protein diets on fat-free mass andmuscle protein synthesis following weight loss:a randomized controlled trial. The FASEB Journal (2013), 27: 3837-3847.

8. BUILD MUSCLE

In order to build muscle or *"bulk up,"* we must consume more than our TDEE. Our goal is to gain as much muscle as possible, while keeping fat gain at the minimum. The more fat we gain, the longer and harder it will take to cut later. As you can see from the above study by Antonio et al., it is possible to gain muscle while losing fat at the same time (1,2). I know this is a difficult statement to understand because you have been taught that you simply cannot gain muscles and lose fat at the same time. I was a firm believer that you cannot do both at the same time until I saw these two studies. How did they accomplish both goals at the same time? The available data showed that if you consume high enough protein and couple it with a progressive resistance training program that focuses on strength gain in addition to a positive energy balance, you can gain lean mass and reduce body fat at the same time. If you are just starting out or coming back from a long lay off from training, this is definitely possible. The subjects in the studies were actually experienced trainers and athletes, so their gains would be harder to achieve (3). Yet, they made the gains, despite conventional wisdom that one cannot gain muscle and lose fat at the same time. The basis of our training program will be based on the exercise selection and centered on strength gain as the study above. The remaining question is how big should our caloric surplus be?

8.1. THE SURPLUS

In a study by Bray et al., subjects consumed in excess of 40% of their baseline energy for 56 days. They were further divided into groups of 5%, 15% and 25% protein diets. What the researchers found was that if the excess energy was from protein, then their sleep and resting 24-hour energy expenditure increased. No changes in fat mass was found and no training regimen was implemented (4). In the study by Antonio et al., participants were consuming an average excess of 378 calories +/- 80 per day with a high protein diet of 3.4 g/kg/day (2). They were also training progressively with heavy weights to gain strength. We can already guess the outcome of this study. The participants gained lean mass while losing body fat. As mentioned previously, the subjects of this study were experienced trainees. In fact, they had about five years of training up their sleeves. How could it be possible that the participants in these studies consumed a rather large surplus, yet did not gain fat? One possible explanation for this might be NEAT, or non-exercise activity thermogenesis. The idea is that we expend energy in any activity that we do, excluding sleep, eating, or sport activities. By doing these activities, we increase our metabolic rate, which varies among different individuals. This variability can be as large as 1000 calories per day (5). Furthermore, protein's thermic effect of feeding or TEF, which is the energy cost of protein metabolism, can account for even higher energy expenditure in subjects consuming higher protein (6). It is possible that when high protein consumption is coupled with a heavy weight training program, NEAT and TEF increased the metabolic rate to compensate for the higher energy consumption.

8.2. BULKING MACROS

In the previous section, we saw that our caloric surplus can be as big as 40% of our total daily dietary calories, as long as our protein consumption is high and our training is consisted of progressive heavy lifting. However, our lives are not under the limited constraint of an experimental study.

Also, a 40% energy intake increase is a lot of foods that we will have to eat. I think it would be better for us to start low and increase as we go along with our bulking. I think a good place to start would be a 10% increase instead. This means that as you gain weight, you will have to recalculate your TDEE and add another 10%, if you want to continue bulking after your goal weight is achieved. For example, if you start at 150 pounds with a TDEE of 2100 calories and end up at 154 pounds and a new TDEE of 2200 calories within 6 weeks of your bulk, you will now have to add 10% to the new TDEE of 2200 calories or 220 calories, if you want to continue bulking after 6 weeks.

Keep your protein consumption at 3.4 g/kg/day, your fat at 30%, and the rest of the calories are for your carbohydrates intake. Let's use our previous example of a 35 years old male, who is 5'5", 170 pounds (77 kg) with a calculated TDEE of 2700 calories for our sample calculation. These are totally made up numbers for calculation practice purposes only. The following unit conversions remain the same.

1 pound = 2.2 kg

1 gram of protein = 4 calories

1 gram of carb = 4 calories

1 gram of fat = 9 calories

8.3. BULKING CALCULATION

We want to create a 10% calories surplus per day. Our TDEE is 2700 calories. So, our total daily dietary calories = 2700 x 1.1 = 2970 calories.

Fat = 2970 calories x (30/100) = 891 calories
Convert fat to grams: 891 calories / (9 calories/g) = 99 grams

Protein = (3.4 g/kg/day) x (170 pounds/2.2 kg/pound) = 263 grams
Convert protein to calories: 263 grams x (4 calories/g) = 1052 calories

Carb = 2970 calories - (891 calories + 1052 calories) = 1027 calories
Convert carb to grams: 1027 calories / (4 calories/g) = 257 grams

So, you would consume 263 grams of protein, 257 grams of carb and 99 grams of fat. Every six to eight weeks, recalculate your TDEE and these calculations once you have gained weight, if you want to continue bulking.

8.4. WHEN TO BULK

This is a common question and is an area of debate. It is a common recommendation that, for men, you can start bulking once you reach 10% body fat or below, and 20% or less for women. At this body fat percentage, you can start gaining slowly to prevent too much fat gain. However, as you can see previously that a surplus as high as 40% when coupled with high protein consumption and heavy weight lifting, you can gain muscle and lose fat at the same time. It is a small, slow fat loss, but fat loss nevertheless. I say let the mirror be your guide. If you are not looking like you have much to lose around the mid section, there is a four pack in there and you are not feeling too great from being in a caloric deficit, you can begin your bulk. I think it might be fine in certain circumstances to begin bulking at 11-12% body fat. How do we know our body fat percentage?

There are many ways of measuring body fat percentage. It would be expensive and I wouldn't want you to have to spend money to find out your number. I think the best method is to look at pictures of what different body fat percentages look like. You can be sure that at 10% body fat percentage or less, there will be visible ab muscles. This is why it is desirable to wait until you get to at least this level of leanness before you start bulking. You will be adding muscles to a lean frame, and, if you need to cut later on, your cut phase will be shorter. You will be looking good all year long. For this reason, I recommend you get to this level of leanness before bulking. You can cut aggressively with a 30% caloric deficit or 500 calories per day, whichever is larger to facilitate faster fat loss. Don't worry about muscle loss as long as you keep your protein consumption high and keep your strength up by lifting heavy weight (1,2,7).

REFERENCES

1. Antonio J. (2014). The effects of consuming a high protein diet (4.4 g/kg/d) on body composition in resistance-trained individuals. JISSN , 11 (19).

2. Antonio J, A. E. (2015). A high protein diet (3.4 g/kg/d) combined with a heavy resistance training program improves body composition in healthy trained men and women – a follow-up investigation. JISSN , 12 (39).

3. American College of Sports Medicine position stand (ACSM).(2009b). Progression models in resistance training for healthyadults. Medicine and Science in Sports and Exercise, 41, 6870708.

4. Bray GA, Redman LM, de Jonge L, Covington J, Rood J, Brock C, et al. (2015). Effect of protein overfeeding on energy expenditure measured in a metabolic chamber. Am J Clin Nutr. 101:496–505.

5. Levine JA, Vander Weg MW, Hill JO, Klesges RC (2006). Non-exercise activity thermogenesis: the crouching tiger hidden dragon of societal weight gain. Arterioscler Thromb Vasc Biol. 26:729–36.

6. Binns A, Gray M, Di Brezzo R (2015). Thermic effect of food, exercise, and total energy expenditure in active females. J Sci Med Sport. 18:204– 8.

7. Pasiakos SM, Cao JJ, Margolis LM, Sauter ER, Whigham LD, McClung JP, Rood JC, Carbone JW, Combs JF, and Young AJ. Effects of high- protein diets on fat-free mass andmuscle protein synthesis following weight loss:a randomized controlled trial. The FASEB Journal (2013), 27: 3837-3847.

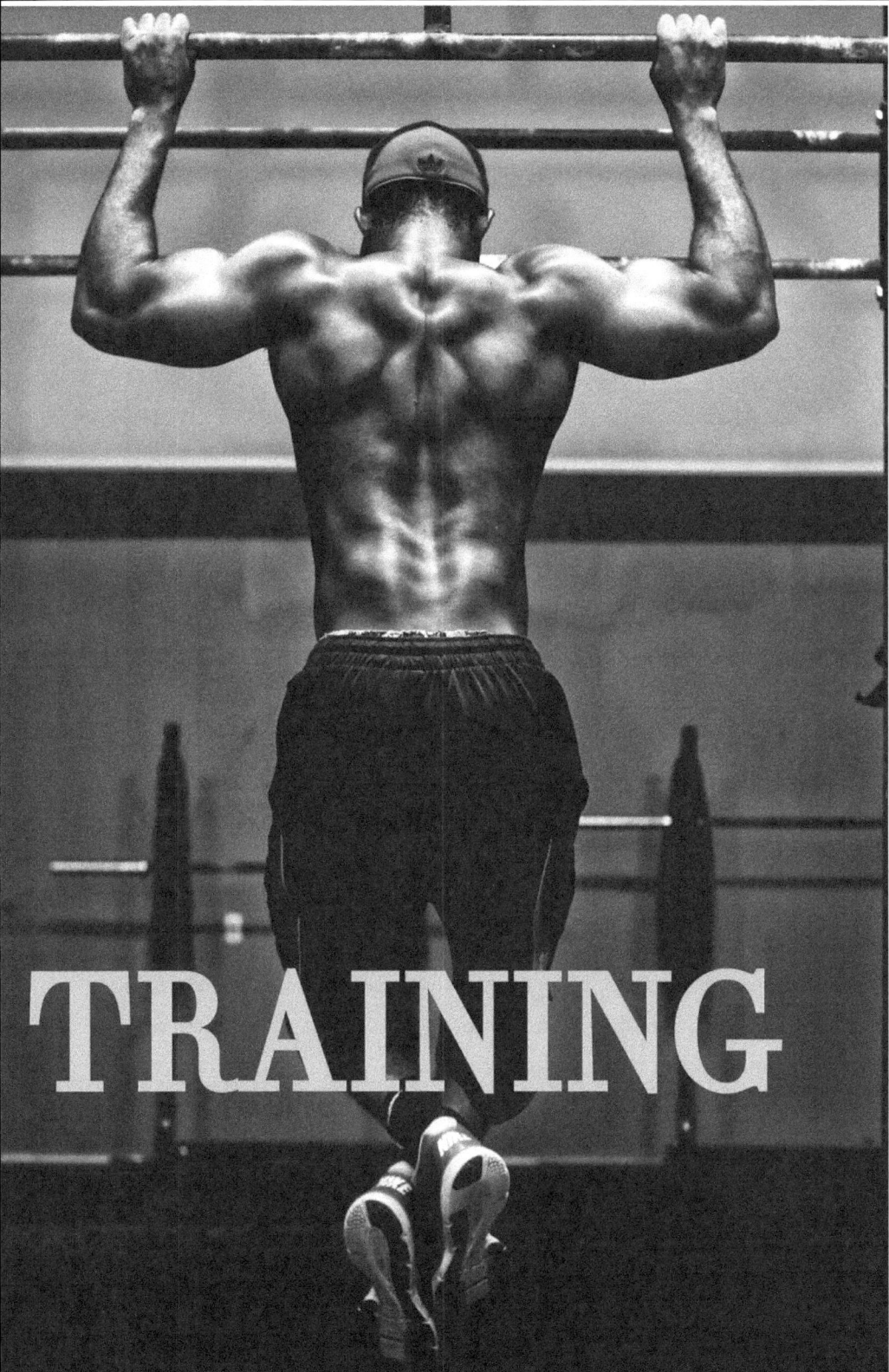

TRAINING

9. ONE MORE TIP

I cannot stress enough the importance of tracking your food consumption via apps like MyFitnessPal, MyPlate or Lifesum. You can also find nutritional information online, but the easiest method would be through apps, which you can download for free. By weighing your foods, you can later estimate its nutritional content when eating out where a balance is not readily available. I understand it is time consuming and you may not have the time to weigh and record your foods. I have a simple solution, but I think it is still important for you to learn about the different portion sizes of different foods. Do learn what a 6 oz piece of chicken, steak, rice, quinoa, or potato looks like. Only then can you use the following method.

The method I am referring to I am sure a lot of you have heard or read about somewhere before. It involves dividing your plate up into three portions of protein, carb, and vegetable (see below). To lose weight, you would reduce your carb portion, but your protein portion would remain the same. To gain weight, you can either increase your carb and/or protein portion. Record your weight to see if you are reaching your goal. If not, reduce your consumption to lose weight or increase it to gain weight. Protein should always remain the same or be increased, but not reduced to keep protein consumption high.

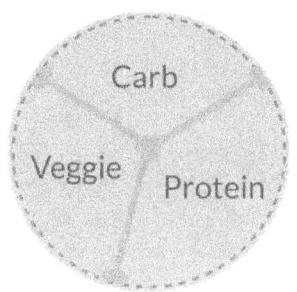

10. TRAINING SCHEME

We will be utilizing compound movements, such as the squat, deadlift, bench press, and overhead press because these movements require a greater amount of neural responses and enable a greater amount of weight to be lifted, and, thus, increase overall muscular strength. It is recommended that novice lifters train 2-3 days per week, intermediate lifters 3-4 days per week, and advanced lifters 4-6 days per week. Using heavy weight of 3-5 reps max have been shown to induce greater strength gain compared to lighter weight that allows for higher reps. Upper/lower body split and total body workouts have similar increases in strength.

However, as one progresses, a higher frequency training schedule that train each muscle group 2-3 times a week is superior to 1 time a week (1).

If you are new to weightlifting or coming back from a long lay off, I would do total body workouts 2-3 days per week. For intermediate lifters, you can either do total body workouts or upper/lower body split 4 days per day. If you are a rare advanced lifter, a body split routine 4-6 days per week is appropriate. As you can see, the popular body split routine of training one or two body parts per day is not for everyone. This routine is reserved for advanced lifters. For the average lifters, a total body routine or upper/lower body routine is recommended. Lifters are classified based on the amount of weight they can lift for the four compound movements mentioned above. The novice lifter's load is typically less than their body weight. The intermediate lifters can typically lift 1-1.5 times their body weight. Advanced lifters load typically falls in the range of 2-3 times their body weight. Keep in mind that these are just arbitrary numbers.

Why the focus on strength? There are primarily three factors that are believed to induce muscular hypertrophy. They are mechanical tension, muscular damage and metabolic stress. Resistance training induces tension in the muscle via the lengthening and disruption of the muscle that leads to a cascade of events that enhance the hypertrophy response. Muscle damage is thought to cause muscular hypertrophy via the inflammatory processes similar to an infection. When the body senses damage, it releases inflammatory mediators to the site that lead to releases of growth factors that regulate cell growth. Metabolic stress refers to the buildup of metabolites, such as lactate, free radicals, hydrogen ions, inorganic phosphates, and others, as a result of training methods that use anaerobic glycolysis for energy. Such training methods include super-set, rest-pause and drop sets. The idea is that after performing an exercise to failure, you don't stop. Instead, you either move immediately to another exercise or reduce weights and perform the same exercise again. By keep going when the muscle is fatigue, it forces your body to turn to anaerobic glycolysis for energy production, and in so doing, metabolites are generated that can lead to increases in muscle fiber degradation and hypertrophy (2). While muscular damage and metabolic stress contribute to muscular hypertrophy, mechanical tension is the single most important factor and is essential to increase muscle mass. As a result, we need to progressively overload the muscle with tension. The best way to do that is to add more weight to the bar as much as possible.

We can also increase the amount of reps. However, as we can see previously the rep range of 3-5 is the best rep range for strength and lean mass gain, while higher rep range is more for endurance (1).

10.1. INSTRUCTIONS

If you are a beginner, pick the three days split. At this stage, your goal is to learn how to do the exercises properly, build stamina, recover, and progress without injuring yourself. For intermediate lifters, pick the four days split. At this stage, you have a solid foundation to build upon. Your goal is to build on your strength to achieve greater muscle mass. Gains are harder for advanced lifters to achieve. You will need to train with focus and determination. Periodization is important for advanced lifters, but the single most important factor is still progressive overload with heavy lifting. The goal for all is to lift as heavy as possible in the range of 3-5 reps. Your goal is to be able to put up more weight as much as possible. As soon as you reach 5 reps in any set, increase the weight by 5-10 pounds. Here is a typical workout set up:

Warm up: Start with a weight you can lift for 12 reps, but only do 5 reps. Increase the weight to a weight you can do 8 reps, but only do 2 reps. Increase the weight again to a weight you can do 6 reps, but only do 1 rep. The point is don't over extend yourself during warm up.

Working sets*: After the warm up, you will be working with the weight you can do 3-5 reps. You will be doing 3-4 working sets per exercise. If you are able to do 5 reps in any exercise, increase the weight by 5-10 pounds. If you are unable to do 3 reps after the increase, then decrease the weight back down and don't add weight until you are able to do 5 reps of the exercise for 3 consecutive sets. Rest for 1-3 minutes between sets.

Note that warm up sets are not part of working sets.

REFERENCES

1. Ratamess NA, Alvar BA, Evetoch TK, Housh TJ, Kibler WB, Kraemer WJ and Triplett NT. Progression models in resistance training for healthy adults. American College of Sports Medicine - Position Stand (2009). 41(3): 687-708.

2. Schoenfeld BJ. The mechanisms of muscle hypertrophy and their application to resistance training. Journal of strength and conditioning research (2010). 24(10): 2857- 2872.

THE SPLIT

TOTAL BODY (3 DAYS)

Day 1:

Barbell Military
Press Squat
Chin up or supinated
pulldown Lying tricep
extension Standing calf raise
Abs for 10 minutes

Day 2:

Deadlift Seated cable row
Floor press
Dumbbell Hammer Curl
Close-grip bench press
Leg Press calf raise
Abs for 10 minutes

Day 3:

Barbell bent-over row
Bench press
Romanian deadlift
Dumbbell lateral raise
Barbell bicep curl
Tricep pressdown
Abs for 10 minutes

TOTAL BODY (4 DAYS)

Day 1:

Barbell bent-over row
Bench press
Incline dumbbell press
Lateral pulldown
Dumbbell lateral raise
Dumbbell biceps curl
Cable triceps pressdown

Day 2:

Deadlift
Leg press
Bulgarian split squat
Standing calf raise
Hip Thrust
Abs for 10 minutes

Day 3:

Barbell military press
Pullups or Chinups
Seated Cable row or
Dumbbell row
Barbell floor press
Cable chest flyes
Barbell bicep curls
Lying tricep extension

Day 4:

Squat
Barbell reverse lunge
Romanian deadlift
Seated calf raise
Lying leg curl
Abs for 10 minutes

BODY SPLIT (5 DAYS)

Day 1:

Bench press Incline Bench press
Dumbbell bench or Decline bench press
Cable crossover
Triceps pressdown

Day 2:

Deadlift
Pull-up or Lateral pulldown
Barbell bent-over row
Standing calf raise
Abs for 10 minutes

Day 3:

Barbell military press
Arnold press
Dumbbell lateral raise
Dumbbell bent-over raise
External rotations

Day 4:

Squat
Leg press
Stiff-leg deadlift
Lying leg curl
Seated calf raise

Day 5:

Close-grip bench press
Barbell curl
Lying triceps extension
Dumbbell hammer curl
Shrugs
Internal rotations
Abs for 10 minutes

10.3. DELOAD

Be sure to back off from hard training every 6 to 8 weeks to allow your body to reset. You can choose to deload more frequently, if you feel fatigue, can't seem to recover, can't sleep, or unable to remain focused during your training. It might be hard for some to accept this, but deload is necessary for you to come back stronger. A week is not going to cause you to lose any muscle or slow down your progress. You will be amazed how good it feels when you do come back full speed again after deloading. So, go ahead and pick any of the options below for deloading for one full week. You can schedule your deloading week to occur during your vacation or business trip when a gym might not be accessible.

Option one: Stay away from the gym for one full week.
Option two: Only lift up to 80% of your 1 rep max for one full week.
Option three: My favorite deloading method is by Chad Waterbury. He recommends starting with a weight you can lift for 12-14 reps, but will only perform 3 reps and keep adding weight to your load by 5% until you reach your 3 rep max load. Note that you will only perform 3 reps on all sets. Rest 1-3 minutes between each set. Take a day off between each day.

Deload Day 1: Squat, Bench press, Lying tricep extension
Deload Day 2: Deadlift, Chinup or pulldown, Hammer Curl
Deload Day 3: Front squat, Barbell military press, Dip
Deload Day 4: Block Deadlift, Seated row, Barbell biceps curl.

That's it! Enjoy your week and eat up to your TDEE. Focus on coming back stronger than ever. Your body and soul will thank you for it.

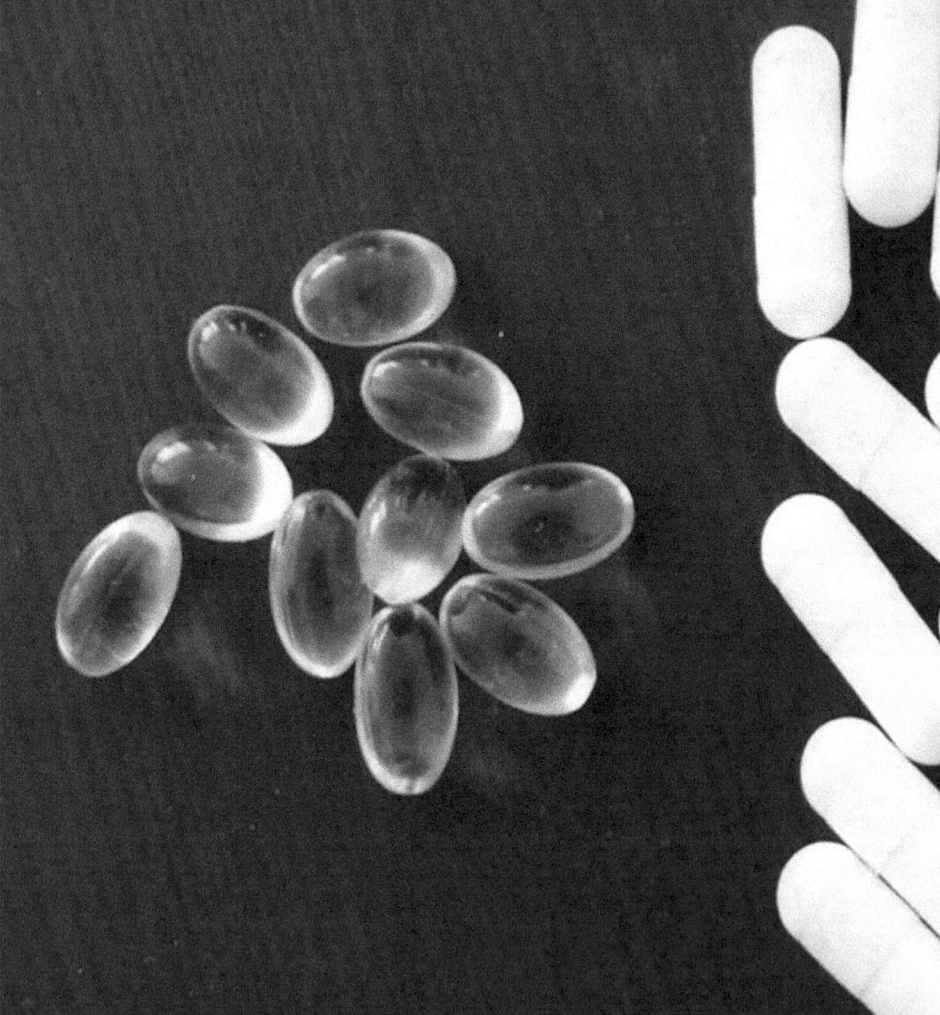

SUPPLEMENTS

11. SUPPLEMENTS

Have you been to a health store that sells natural health products lately? Have you done a search on the benefits of Beta-hydroxy-beta-methylbutyric acid before? Many would have you believe that you had better jump on their supplements right away, if you are to have any hope of building muscle, lose fat, or lead a healthy lifestyle the "natural" way. In order for me to jump on any supplements, I want to know the answers to two important questions. Firstly, what is it alleged benefits? Secondly, are there any scientific facts to back the claim? I don't just want evidence to prove its benefits from sub-par studies conducted by the manufacturers of the products themselves. I want succinctly concrete, third-party independent, reputable, and replicable scientific data that is free of bias and commercial benefits. I want the data to be published in a reputable peer-reviewed journal also. Even when all these things checked out, I want to make sure the products I am putting into my body, you know the one I spend countless of hours in the gym and outside of the gym trying to nourish it with proper nutrition, are produced in an FDA-approved facility using quality ingredients. We should demand the best and nothing, but the best. I cannot possibly go over every single supplement out there because there are just simply too many of them for the scope of this book. Instead I will go over the ones I think are beneficial and have scientific data to back them up in our quest to build muscle and lose fat. I will go over the different schemes that people employ to try to get more money out of you or sell you an inferior product.

11.1. WHEY PROTEIN

Whey is a liquid that is left over during cheese production. When rennin, a protein-digesting enzyme found in the stomach of young cows, sheep, or goats, is added to milk during cheese making, whey and casein separates. Whey is a fast digesting protein, while casein is slow-digesting. Both are considered high quality proteins and aid in muscle protein synthesis. The initial liquid is called *whey protein concentrate*, which contains about 80% proteins and the rest contains carbohydrates and fats. *Whey protein isolates* are whey protein concentrate that have been filtered further to yield about 90-95% protein by weight. Thus, whey protein isolates have a higher protein concentration and less carbohydrates and fats. *Whey protein hydrolysate* is whey protein isolates that have been pre- digested for even faster absorption. In term of cost, whey protein concentrate is the cheapest, then whey protein isolates is more costly, and whey protein hydrolysate is the most expensive.

Why is whey protein important? It have been shown to increase muscle protein synthesis, especially when coupled with exercise (1,2,3). Which form of whey protein is superior? All forms of whey protein contain essential amino acids. Therefore, they are equally efficacious. However, if you are looking to reduce carbohydrates and fats, whey protein isolates have less carbohydrates and fats content that might be more suitable for you. I personally prefer whey protein isolates for this reason. That leads us to the next question. Are all brands of whey proteins created equal? When deciding which brand to buy, I take into account purity and cost. First, I look at the label to see how many grams of protein are contained in each serving or scoop provided. If the protein content is almost as big as the serving or scoop size, then I can be sure that the product does not contain much fillers, artificial sweetener or flavor. The two should be of the same size for this reason. For example, if the protein content per serving or scoop is 25 grams, then the serving or scoop size should be around 28 grams. If you see the serving or scoop size is much larger than the protein content, then you know there are other inactive ingredients being added to the product. The more closely the two sizes match up in weight, the more pure the product. The other purity consideration I want to look out for is the types of proteins being packaged in the product. I want whey protein isolates, so I would choose a product that contains just whey protein isolates and nothing else. There are products that contain a blend of different whey proteins, such as concentrate, isolates, egg, milk proteins, or branched chain amino acids (BCAA). The cheaper proteins and/or BCAA are being thrown in to lower manufacturing cost, yet advertised as whey protein isolates. Look for products that contain only whey protein isolates. There is nothing wrong with blended products. I would prefer to spend my money on products that will give me more proteins content, less carbs and fats, and lower in calories. Lastly, I look at cost. I know it is cliche, but you get what you pay for. If two products are being equal, but one is much cheaper than the other, then I would rather buy the one that is a bit more expensive. Making whey proteins is time consuming and costly. Therefore, pricing should be relatively the same across different brands. We are left with whey protein hydrolysate, which is not superior to whey protein isolates. Despite their superior absorption, they have not been found to be superior at inducing muscle protein synthesis.

Casein protein, the other by-product of cheese making, is inferior to whey protein due to its essential amino acid profile, which have been shown to jump start muscle protein synthesis, particularly leucine (4,5). They are also harder to mix and more constipating. However, they are slow digesting and due to this property casein is usually taken at night to provide for a constant supply of amino acids while you sleep. Since casein is not superior to whey protein, I prefer not to have to add it to my medicine cabinet. Remember total daily protein consumption is what matters most. Protein powder is meant to be used as a supplement. So, use the one that you are most comfortable with in term of purity, taste, effectiveness and cost. It is more important to choose the one that you are more willing to take to help you reach your goal.

11.2. CREATINE

Creatine is a natural compound found in the muscle, brain, kidney and liver. When it is stored in the muscle, it is phosphorylated to phosphocreatine. It serves as a phosphate ion reserve that is used to convert ADP into ATP, which is the energy molecule the body uses. During exercise, our body breaks ATP (contains 3 phosphate ions) down to ADP (contains 2 phosphate ions). Phosphocreatine donates a phosphate ion to convert ADP back to ATP. Thus, creatine intake can increase energy stores, which is depleted during physical activities. Creatine have been found to increase lean mass, strength, and power output (6). The mechanisms of how creatine is able to help attain gain in lean mass, strength, and power output is still unknown. We do know that creatine affects cellular hydration status, which have been shown to affect protein metabolism. Some studies have shown that creatine decreases protein breakdown rate, especially leucine breakdown rate. Some studies also suggest that creatine increases the amount of work to be performed, and, thus, indirectly increases lean mass, which leads to gain in strength and power output as a result (7). Nevertheless, it is becoming clear that creatine supplementation has multiple benefits without any clinically significant side effects. Most side effects are gastrointestinal in nature, such as stomach upset and cramping (8). These side effects can be mitigated by adequate hydration and slower consumption by drinking it slowly rather than chugging it down with one sip. Creatine does not cause kidney issues, as previously thought.

11.3. VITAMIN D

Vitamin D is an essential fat-soluble micronutrient that is made from cholesterol. However, our body needs the UV ray from the sun in order to produce vitamin D. Deficiency have been shown to be linked to increased body fat and decreased strength. Gilsanz et al. noted in a study that women who were deficient in vitamin D had a 24% increase in muscle tissue fat infiltration compared to women who had normal level, and muscle tissue fat infiltration have been associated with decreased strength and power output (9). Carrillo et al. did a study in which subjects were given 4000 IU of vitamin D daily versus placebo. Both groups did resistance training, as well as treadmill work, and their diets were controlled for similar caloric and macronutrients intake. The results show increase in power output and reduced waist circumference (10). In another study that was conducted to investigate vitamin D's role in muscle recovery, repair, regeneration and hypertrophy, participants were given 4000 IU daily. Their right quadriceps muscle was damaged via leg extensions. After six weeks, Owens et al. found that supplementation of vitamin D resulted in improved muscle recovery 48 hours and 7 days post exercise (11). Vitamin D also have other benefits that are beneficial to your health, such as bone health, improved immune function and cognition, as well as reduction in risks of cancer, heart disease and diabetes to name a few. In light of these benefits, it is absolutely essential to pay attention to your vitamin D level. You can have it checked at your doctor's office via a simple blood test. Most people don't have optimal level, so oral supplementation is necessary.

11.4. FISH OIL

Fish oil is rich in Omega-3 fatty acids. The two Omega-3 fatty acids that are of most importance are eicosapentaenoic acid (EPA) and docosahexaenoic acid (DHA). They are thought to have many health benefits, but most of these benefits were derived from animal studies and have been inconsistent in human trials. Recently, a meta-analysis was done to investigate the anti-obesity effects of fish oil with or without lifestyle modification. Du et al. concluded that fish oil is beneficial in the reduction of abdominal fat, especially with a weight loss program (12). It is thought that Omega-3 fatty acids achieve abdominal fat reduction by inducing lipogenic gene down regulation, changes in lipid synthesis or storage. There is also evidence that fish oil reduces the hard to target visceral fat. For this reason, I recommend supplementation with fish oil. The American Heart Association recommends one gram of fish oil per day. Visceral fat is difficult to burn, so anything that can help target visceral fat will be beneficial to our health in the long term. By reducing abdominal fat, it might also reduce our risk of the metabolic syndrome that is often associated with the development of diabetes and heart disease.

11.5. HOW TO TAKE

Whey Protein: Take it as a supplement to meet your total daily protein intake, but no more than 50% of your total daily protein requirement should come from powder protein. If you haven't had anything to eat for three or more hours prior to training, have your protein shake immediately after your training session within 30 minutes. If you ate something within three hours prior to training, you can have your protein shake within 2 hours. The anabolic window is over-exaggerated. Muscle protein synthesis is elevated for 24 hours after your training session. There is no need to run home to gulp down your protein shake, if you already had some protein from food prior to training. Total daily protein intake is more important than when it is consumed. Ideally, protein consumption should be spread out every 3-4 hours throughout the day while awake.

Creatine: Take 5 grams of creatine monohydrate every day. Creatine is not time-dependent, so you can have it at any time in the day. Creatine monohydrate is the most well studied form of creatine and is the cheapest. No need to use the more expensive version, creatine hydrochloride or HCL.

Vitamin D: Take vitamin D3 (cholecalciferol) 4000 IU per day with food, preferably with fat. You can take it together with your fish oil.

Fish oil: Take 1 gram of fish oil per day. Make sure it contains at least 250- 500 mg of EPA/DHA combined.

Consult with your physician before starting any supplement, as they may interact with your medical conditions or medications.

REFERENCES

1. Biogolo G1, Tipton KD, Klein S, Wolfe RR. An abundant supply of amino acids enhances the metabolic effect of exercise on muscle protein. Am J Physiol. (1997) Jul;273(1 Pt 1):E122-9.

2. Farnfield MM, Breen L, Carey KA, Garnham A, Cameron-Smith A. Activation of mTOR signalling in young and old human skeletal muscle in response to combined resistance exercise and whey protein ingestion. Applied Physiology, Nutrition, and Metabolism. (2012). 37:21-30.

3. Burd NA, West DW, Moore DR, Atherton PJ, Staples AW, Prior T, Tang JE, Rennie MJ, Baker SK, Phillips SM. Enhanced amino acid sensitivity of myofibrillar protein synthesis persists for up to 24 h after resistance exercise in young men. J Nutr. (2011) Apr 1;141(4):568-73.

4. Dangin M, Boirie Y, Guillet C, Beaufrère B. Influence of the protein digestion rate on protein turnover in young and elderly subjects. J Nutr. (2002) Oct;132(10):3228S-33S.

5. Norton LE, Layman DK, Bunpo P, Anthony TG, Brana DV, Garlick PJ. The leucine content of a complete meal directs peak activation but not duration of skeletal muscle protein synthesis and mammalian target of rapamycin signaling in rats. J Nutr. (2009) Jun;139(6):1103-9.

6. Wyss M, Kaddurah-Daouk R. Creatine and creatinine metabolism. Physiol Rev. (2000) Jul;80(3):1107-213.

7. Parise G, Mihic S, Maclennan D, Yarasheski KE, Tarnopolsky MA. Effects of acute creatine monohydrate supplementationon leucine kinetics and mixed-muscle protein synthesis. J Appl Physiol (2001) 91: 1041–1047.

8. Groeneveld GJ, Beijer C, Veldink JH, Kalmijn S, Wokke JH, van den Berg LH. Few adverse effects of long-term creatine supplementation in a placebo-controlled trial. Int J Sports Med. (2005) May; 26(4):307-13.

9. Gilsanz V, Kremer A, Mo AO, Wren TA, Kremer R. Vitamin D status and its relation to muscle mass and muscle fat in young women. J Clin Endocrinol Metab. (2010); 95(4):1595–1601.

10. Carrillo AE, Flynn MG, Pinkston C, Markofski MM, Jiang Y, Donkin SS, Teegarden D. Impact of vitamin D supplementation during a resistance training intervention on body composition, muscle function, and glucose tolerance in overweight and obese adults. Clin Nutr. (2013) June ; 32(3): 375–381.

11. Owens DJ, Sharples AP, Polydorou I, Alwan N, Donovan T, Tang J, Fraser WD, Cooper RG, Morton JP, Stewart C, Close GL. A systems based investigation into vitamin D and skeletal muscle repair, regeneration,and hypertrophy. Am J Physiol Endocrinol Metab. (2015) 309: E1019– E1031.

12. Du S, Jin J, Fang W, Su Q. Does Fish Oil Have an Anti-Obesity Effect in Overweight/Obese Adults? A Meta-Analysisof Randomized Controlled Trials. PLoS ONE. (2015) 10(11): e0142652.

SUMMARY

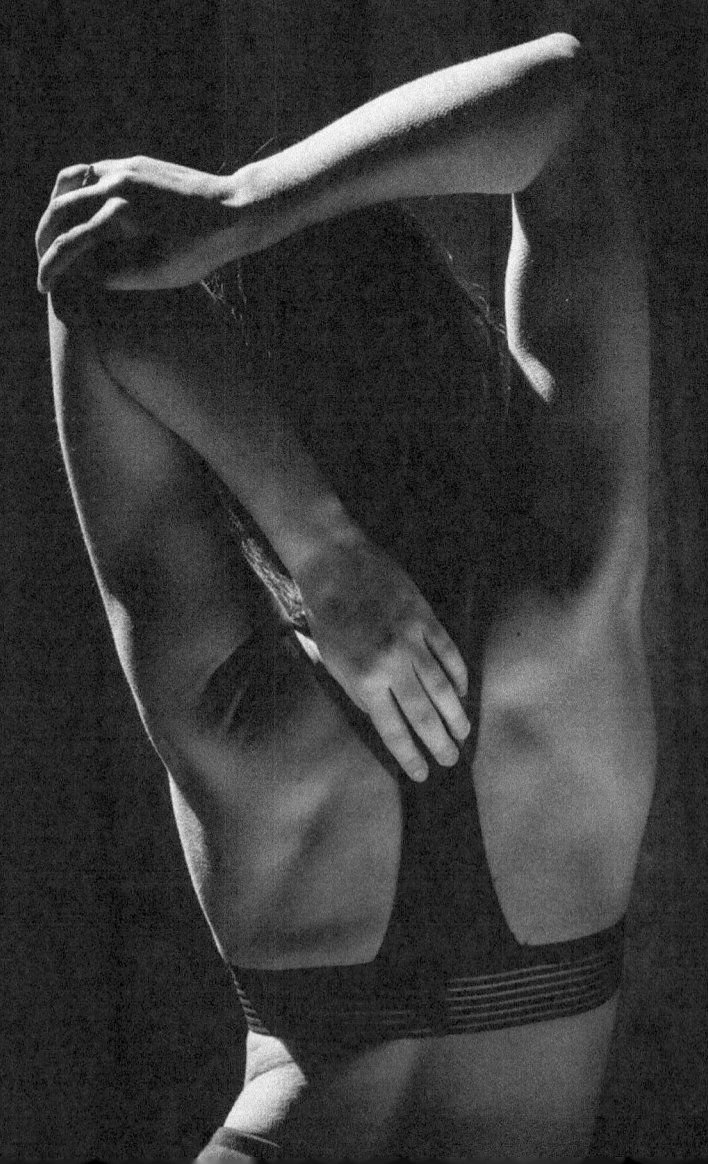

12. SUMMARY

1. Energy balance (caloric intake) is what determines whether you gain or lose weight. If the energy balance is positive, energy taken in is greater than energy used, and you gain weight. On the contrary, if the energy balance is negative, then you lose weight.

2. Estimate your TDEE to find out your total daily dietary calories needed to maintain weight.

3. Weigh yourself every day for two weeks, calculate the average of your weight every week to see if you are gaining or losing weight while eating up to your TDEE.

4. To lose weight, consume less than your TDEE. Your caloric deficit can be as large as 30% of your TDEE. Your total daily dietary calories is your TDEE - 30% or TDEE - [TDEE x (30/100)]. During your CUT, your macros are as follows, 20% fat, protein is 3.4 g/kg/day, and carbs are the rest of the calories.

5. To gain weight, consume more than your TDEE. Your caloric surplus can be as large as 40% of your TDEE. Your total daily dietary calories is your TDEE + 40% or TDEE + [TDEE x (40/100)]. During your BULK, your macros are as follows, 30% fat, protein is 3.4 g/kg/day, and carbs are the rest of the calories.

6. Keep protein consumption high while cutting weight to avoid lean body mass loss. If you don't, you will lose both fat and muscle, which will reduce you to being "skinny fat."

7. Keep your caloric surplus small and increase as you go to keep fat gain at minimum.

8. Last, but not least, if you haven't seen the research results already...

KEEP YOUR PROTEIN INTAKE HIGH,

LIFT HEAVY
and
PUT UP MORE
WEIGHT ON THE BAR
AS OFTEN AS
POSSIBLE IN THE GYM!!!